Table of Contents

# INTRODUCTION

Epilepsy is a neurological condition that causes unprovoked, recurrent seizures. A seizure is a sudden rush of abnormal electrical activity in your brain. Doctors diagnose epilepsy when you have two or more seizures with no other identifiable cause. Epilepsy affects 50 millionpeople around the world, according to the World Health Organization (WHO) and nearly 3.5 million people in the United States, per the Centers for Disease Control and Prevention (CDC). Anyone can develop epilepsy, but it most commonlyonsets in young children and older adults. According to research published in 2021, men develop epilepsy more often than women, possibly because of higher exposure to risk factors like alcohol use and head trauma. The two main types of seizures are:

generalized seizures

focal seizures

# What are the symptoms of epilepsy?

Seizures are the main symptom of epilepsy. Symptoms differ from person to person and according to the type of seizure.

Focal (partial) seizures

A focal aware seizure (previously called simple partial seizure) does not involve loss of consciousness. Symptoms include:

alterations to sense of taste, smell, sight, hearing, or touch

dizziness

tingling and twitching of limbs

Focal unaware seizures (previously called complex partial seizures) involve loss of awareness or consciousness. Other symptoms include:

staring blankly

unresponsiveness

performing repetitive movements

Generalized seizures

Generalized seizures involve the whole brain. Subtypes include:

Absence seizures. Absence seizures used to be called "petit mal seizures." They tend to cause a short loss of awareness, a blank stare, and may cause repetitive movements like lip smacking or blinking.

Tonic seizures. Tonic seizures cause sudden stiffness in the muscles in your legs, arms, or trunk.

Atonic seizures. Atonic seizures lead to loss of muscle control. They're also called "drop seizures" because a sudden loss of muscle strength can make you fall suddenly.

Clonic seizures. Clonic seizures are characterized by repeated, jerky muscle movements of the face, neck, and arms.

Myoclonic seizures. Myoclonic seizures cause spontaneous quick twitching of the arms and legs. Sometimes these seizures cluster together.

Tonic-clonic seizures. Tonic-clonic seizures used to be called "grand mal seizures." Symptoms include:

stiffening of the body

shaking

loss of bladder or bowel control

biting of the tongue

loss of consciousness

Following a seizure, you may not remember having one, or you might feel slightly ill for a few hours.


First aid for seizures

It's important to note that most seizures don't require emergency medical attention, and you can't stop a seizure once it's in progress.

When you're with somebody having a mild seizure:

Stay with the person until their seizure ends and they're awake.

Once they're awake, guide them to a safe place and tell them what happen.

Stay calm and try to keep other people calm.

Speak calmly.

Check for a medical bracelet.

Offer to help the person get home safely.

If the person is having a tonic-clonic seizure, which causes uncontrolled shaking or jerking:

Ease the person to the ground.

Turn them gently onto their side to help them breathe.

Clear any dangerous objects away from them.

Put something soft under their head.

If they wear glasses, remove them.

Loosen any clothing, such as a tie, that may affect breathing.

Time the seizure and call 911 if it lasts longer than 5 minutesTrusted Source.

When someone is having a seizure, it's critical to never:

hold the person down or try to stop their movements

put anything in their mouth

give them mouth to mouth

offer the person food or water until they're fully alert

Learn more about epilepsy first aid.

## What causes epilepsy?

In about half of people with epilepsyTrusted Source, the cause cannot be determined, per the WHO. A variety of factors can contribute to the development of seizures, such as:

traumatic brain injury or other head trauma

brain scarring after a brain injury (post-traumatic epilepsy)

serious illness or very high fever

stroke, which causes about halfTrusted Source of epilepsy cases in older adults when there's no identifiable cause, according to the CDC

lack of oxygen to the brain

brain tumor or cyst

dementia, including Alzheimer's disease

maternal use of some drugs, prenatal injury, brain malformation, or lack of oxygen at birth

infectious conditions like HIV and AIDS and meningitis

genetic or developmental disorders or neurological diseases

Epilepsy can develop at any age, but diagnosis usually occurs in early childhood or after 60 years old.

*Researchers first identified genes linked to epilepsy in the late 1990s, according to the Epilepsy Foundation. Since then, they Is epilepsy hereditary?*
have discovered more than 500 genesTrusted Source thought to contribute to its development. Some genes are associated with certain types of epilepsy. For example, people with Dravet syndrome often have abnormal changes in their SCN1A gene. Not all genes linked to epilepsy are passed down through families. Some gene mutations develop in children even if they're not present in either parent. These are called "de novo mutations." Some types of epilepsy are more common in people with a family history, but most children of people with epilepsy don't develop epilepsy themselves. According to the Epilepsy Foundation, even if a child has a parent or sibling with epilepsy, the chances that they'll develop the condition by age 40 is still less than 5 percent.

The chances of developing epilepsy are higher if a close relative has a generalized epilepsy rather than a focal epilepsy. If your parent has epilepsy due to another cause, such as stroke or brain injury, it does not affect your chances of developing seizures. Certain rare conditions, such as tuberous sclerosis and neurofibromatosis, can cause seizures. These conditions can run in families. Genetics may also make some people more susceptible to seizures from environmental triggers. If you have epilepsy and are concerned about starting a family, consider arranging a consultation with a genetic counselor.

What triggers an epileptic seizure?

Some people identify things or situations that trigger their seizures. A few of the most common known triggers are:

lack of sleep

illness or fever

stress

bright lights, flashing lights, or patterns

caffeine, alcohol or alcohol withdrawal, medications, or illegal drugs skipping meals, overeating, or specific food ingredients

very low blood sugar

head injury

Identifying triggers isn't always easy. A single incident doesn't always mean something is a trigger. Often, a combination of factors triggers a seizure. A good way to find your triggers is to keep a seizure journal. After each seizure, note the following:

day and time

what activity you were involved in

what was happening around you

unusual sights, smells, or sounds

unusual stressors

what you were eating or how long it had been since you'd eaten

your level of fatigue and how well you slept the night before

You can also use your seizure journal to determine if your medications are working. Note how you felt just before and just after your seizure, and any side effects. Bring the journal with you when you visit the doctor. It may be useful for your doctor if adjusting your medications or exploring other treatments is, or becomes, necessary.

*Potential complications of epilepsy*
Epileptic seizures disrupt the electrical activity of your brain, which can directly or indirectly affect many parts of your body. Potential complications of epilepsy include:

injury from falling during a seizure

injury while operating an automobile or machinery

depression

brain damage from prolonged and uncontrolled seizures

choking on food or saliva

medication side effects

Each year, about 1.16 out of every 1,000 peopleTrusted Source with epilepsy experience sudden unexpected death in epilepsy (SUDEP), according to the CDC. SUDEP is an epilepsy-related death not caused by drowning, injury, or another known cause. Pauses in breathing, airway obstruction, and abnormal heart rhythm are thought to contribute.

SUDEP is more common in people with epilepsy that is not well managed. Taking all your medication as prescribed and visiting your doctor regularly can help you minimize your risk.

## How is epilepsy diagnosed?

If you suspect you've had a seizure, see a doctor as soon as possible. A seizure can be a symptom of a serious medical issue. Your medical history and symptoms will help your doctor decide which tests will be helpful. They'll likely give you a neurological examination to test your motor abilities and mental functioning. To diagnose epilepsy, other conditions that cause seizures should be ruled out. A doctor will probably order a complete blood count (CBC) and chemistry of your blood. Blood tests may be used to look for:

signs of infectious diseases

liver and kidney function

blood glucose levels

Electroencephalogram (EEG) is the most common test used to diagnose epilepsy. It's a noninvasive and painless test that involves placing electrodes on your scalp to search for abnormal patterns in your brain's electrical activity. You may be asked to perform a specific task during the test. In some cases, the test is performed while you sleep. Imaging tests can reveal tumors and other abnormalities that can cause seizures. These tests might include:

CT scan

MRI

positron emission tomography (PET)

single-photon emission computerized tomography

Epilepsy is usually diagnosed if you have seizures, but there's no apparent or reversible cause.

## How is epilepsy treated?

Treatment for epilepsy may help you have fewer seizures or stop seizures completely. Your treatment plan will be based on:

the severity of your symptoms

your health

how well you respond to therapy

Some treatment options include:

Anti-epileptic (anticonvulsant, antiseizure) drugs. Anti-epileptic medications can help reduce the number of seizures you have. In some people, they may eliminate seizures. To be most effective, the medication must be taken exactly as your doctor prescribed.

Vagus nerve stimulator. This device is surgically placed under the skin on your chest and electrically stimulates the nerve that runs through your neck to prevent seizures.

Ketogenic diet. According to the Epilepsy Foundation, more than half of children who do not respond to medications benefit from the ketogenic diet, which is a high fat and low carbohydrate diet.

Brain surgery. The area of the brain that causes seizure activity can be removed or altered if you and your healthcare team determine it's the right treatment for your condition.

Research into new treatments is ongoing. One treatment that may be more widely available in the future is deep brain stimulation. It involves implanting electrodes into your brain and a generator into your chest. The generator sends electrical impulses to your brain to help decrease seizures. The FDA approved the use of deep brain stimulation in 2018 in people over 18 years old with focal onset seizures who have not responded to at least three anti-epileptic medications. Minimally invasive surgeries and radiosurgery are also being investigated.

*Medications for epilepsy*

The first-line treatment for epilepsy is antiseizure medication. These drugs are designed to help reduce the frequency and severity of seizures. They cannot stop a seizure that's already in progress, and they are not a cure for epilepsy. These medications are absorbed by your stomach. They then travel through your bloodstream to your brain. They affect neurotransmitters in a way that reduces the electrical activity that leads to seizures. There are many antiseizure drugs on the market. Your doctor can prescribe a single drug or a combination of drugs, depending on your type of seizure. Common epilepsy medications include:

levetiracetam (Keppra)

lamotrigine (Lamictal)

topiramate (Topamax)

valproic acid (Depakote)

carbamazepine (Tegretol)

ethosuximide (Zarontin)

These medications are generally available in tablet, liquid, or injectable forms and are taken once or twice a day. Your doctor will initially prescribe the lowest possible dose, which can be adjusted until it starts to work. These medications must be taken consistently and as prescribed. Some potential side effects may include:

fatigue

dizziness

skin rash

poor coordination

memory problems

Rare, but serious side effects include depression and inflammation of the liver or other organs. Epilepsy is different for everybody, but in most cases, people see improvement with antiseizure medication. Some children with epilepsy may stop having seizures and can stop taking medication.

*Is surgery an option for epilepsy management?*
If medication can't decrease your number of seizures, another option is brain surgery.

Resection

The most common surgery is resection. This involves removing the part of your brain where the seizures start. Most often, the temporal lobe is removed in a procedure known as temporal lobectomy. In some cases, this can stop seizure activity. In some cases, you'll be kept awake during this surgery so doctors can talk with you and avoid removing part of the brain that controls important functions such as vision, hearing, speech, or movement.

Multiple subpial transection

If the area of the brain is too big or important to remove, surgeons may perform another procedure called a multiple subpial transection, or disconnection. During this procedure, the surgeon makes cuts in your brain to interrupt the nerve pathway. This cut keeps seizures from spreading to other areas of your brain. After surgery, some people are able to cut down on antiseizure medications or even stop taking them, their doctor's oversight. There are risks to any surgery, including a negative reaction to anesthesia, bleeding, and infection. Surgery of the brain can sometimes result in cognitive changes.

It can be a good idea to discuss the pros and cons of the different procedures with your surgeon and other healthcare team members. You may also want to seek a second opinion before making a final decision.


When to contact a doctor

It's important to see your doctor regularly for checkups. People with well-managed epilepsy should consider meeting with their family doctor or epilepsy specialist at least once per year, according to the National Health Service. People with epilepsy that is not well managed may need to see their doctor more often. It's also a good idea to schedule an appointment with your doctor if you experience any new symptoms or if you experience side effects after your medication has been changed.

# LIVING WITH EPILEPSY: WHAT TO EXPECT

Epilepsy is a chronic disorder that can affect many parts of your life. Laws vary from state to state, but if your seizures are not well managed, you may not be allowed to drive. Because you never know when a seizure will occur, many everyday activities like crossing a busy street can become dangerous. These problems can lead to loss of independence. In addition to regular doctor visits and following your treatment plan, here are some things you can do to cope:

Keep a seizure diary to help identify possible triggers so you can avoid them.

Wear a medical alert bracelet to let people know that you have epilepsy so you get the right medical help if you have a seizure and can't speak.

Teach the people closest to you about seizures and what to do in an emergency.

Seek professional help if you have — or think you have — symptoms of depression or anxiety.

Join a support group for people with seizure disorders.

Engage in health-promoting activities like eating a nutrient-rich, balanced diet and getting regular exercise.

## Is there a cure for epilepsy?

Early treatment with medication can help reduce seizure frequency and the chances of serious complications. Epilepsy surgery, meanwhile, is considered curative in most cases. Approximately 30 percentTrusted Source of people with partial epilepsy and 25 percent of people with generalized epilepsy have seizures that don't respond well to medication. If medication fails, your doctor may recommend surgery or vagus nerve stimulation.

Two types of brain surgery can cut down on or eliminate seizures. One type, called resection, involves removing the part of the brain where seizures originate. When the area of the brain responsible for seizures is too vital or large to remove, the surgeon can perform a disconnection. This involves interrupting the nerve pathway by making cuts in the brain. This keeps seizures from spreading to other parts of the brain. Dozens of other avenues of research into the causes, treatment, and potential cures for epilepsy are ongoing. Although there's no cure at this time, the right treatment can result in a dramatic improvement in your condition and your quality of life.

*Facts and statistics about epilepsy*
Worldwide, 50 million people have epilepsy. In the United States, about 3 million people and 470,000 children have epilepsy and about 150,000 new cases are diagnosed each year.

As many as 500 genesTrusted Source may relate to epilepsy in some way.

Strokes cause about halfTrusted Source of cases of epilepsy in older adults when there is no other identifiable cause.

About 40 percent of U.S. children with epilepsy between 4 and 15 years old have another neurological disorder. The most common are intellectual disability, speech-language disability, or specific learning disabilities.

About 1.9 percent of epilepsy-related deaths in the United States are due to prolonged seizures, a condition known as status epilepticus.

Seizures start in people over 65 years old almost as often as they start in children.

More than 1 million people in the United States have epilepsy that is not well managed.

About 80 percentTrusted Source of people with epilepsy live in low income countries and don't receive proper treatment.

The cause of epilepsy is unknown about half of cases worldwideTrusted Source.

Learn more facts and statistics about epilepsy.

## What Causes Dizziness and How to Treat It

Possible causes of dizziness include vertigo, dehydration, hypoglycemia, and neurological conditions. Lifestyle changes and medications are among the most common treatments. Dizziness is the feeling of being lightheaded, woozy, or off-balance. It's linked to the sensory organs, specifically the eyes and ears, so it can sometimes cause fainting. Dizziness isn't a disease itself but rather a symptom of various disorders.

Dizziness is common. Occasional dizziness isn't something to worry about. However, it's important to call a doctor immediately if you're experiencing repeated episodes of dizziness for no apparent reason or for a prolonged period.

*Dizziness causes*
Dizziness has a variety of possible causes.

Vertigo and disequilibrium

True dizziness is the feeling of lightheadedness or nearly fainting. Vertigo and disequilibrium may both cause a feeling of dizziness, but these two terms describe distinct sensations. Vertigo is characterized by a spinning sensation, like the room is moving. It may also feel like motion sickness or as if you're leaning to one side. Disequilibrium is a loss of balance or equilibrium.

A common cause of vertigo and vertigo-related dizziness is benign positional vertigo (BPV). BPV leads to short-term dizziness when someone changes positions quickly, such as sitting up in bed after lying down. Dizziness and vertigo can also be triggered by Meniere's disease. This condition causes fluid to build up in the ear with associated ear fullness, hearing loss, and tinnitus. Another possible cause of dizziness and vertigo is an acoustic neuroma. This noncancerous tumor forms on the vestibulocochlear nerve (auditory nerve), which connects the inner ear to the brain.

Common causes

Losing too much fluid can result in dehydration, one of the most common causes of dizziness. Symptoms of dehydration include thirst and dry skin.

Other common causes of dizziness include a migraine attack or alcohol.

Dizziness can also result from a problem in the inner ear, which is the area that senses movement and regulates balance. These problems include hearing loss. Dizziness may be linked to certain medications, too, including:

muscle relaxants

antiepileptic drugs

antihistamines

blood pressure medications

Other possible causes

Some other potential causes of dizziness include:

Sudden drop in blood pressure: Sudden low blood pressure may be caused by various medical conditions or even from standing up (orthostatic hypotension). It can lead to dizziness and falling, especially in older adults.

Cardiomyopathy: In this condition, the heart muscles become rigid and weak and pump less blood. Symptoms can include dizziness, fainting, and trouble breathing.

Heart attack: While chest pain is the most common indicator of a heart attack, dizziness or lightheadedness can also be symptoms. They occur if there's not enough blood reaching your brain.

Arrhythmia: Arrhythmia occurs when the heart beats at an atypical pace. It can cause dizziness, lightheadedness, or shortness of breath.

Circulation problems: Cardiomyopathy, heart attack, and other heart conditions can result in circulation problems, where your heart is unable to pump enough blood. This can cause you to feel dizzy.

Excessive exercise: Overexerting yourself may make you feel dizzy or lightheaded. It can also lead to dehydration and heat exhaustion, which can both cause dizziness.

Heat exhaustion: If you're in a hot environment and sweating excessively, you're likely experiencing heat exhaustion. The condition may make you feel dizzy, thirsty, and weak.

Decrease in blood volume: Low blood volume can result from bleeding or dehydration. It can cause dizziness, fatigue, and low blood pressure. Learn more about the relationship between dehydration and blood pressure.

Anxiety disorders: Dizziness may be related to anxiety with no other physical causes. You may have repeated episodes of dizziness.

Anemia: Anemia is a low red blood cell count. Low levels of iron-rich hemoglobin in your red blood cells mean the cells can't transport enough oxygen throughout the body. The lack of oxygen caused by anemia may make you feel dizzy, tired, or short of breath.

Hypoglycemia: Hypoglycemia, or low blood sugar, can make you feel shaky, lightheaded, or hungry. Severe hypoglycemia is a serious condition that can cause a seizure. Discover other symptoms associated with hypoglycemia.

Carbon monoxide poisoning: If carbon monoxide fumes from cars, grills, or furnaces build up indoors, breathing them in can be fatal. Dizziness, headache, and vomiting are all symptoms.

Motion sickness: Traveling by car or boat or experiencing other types of motion can give you motion sickness. You may feel dizzy and nauseous.

Multiple sclerosis (MS): Multiple sclerosis (MS) damages the brain and spinal cord. It causes a range of symptoms that can include dizziness.

Parkinson's disease: Dizziness is a common symptom of Parkinson's disease, a neurological condition that causes shaking and balance issues. Dizziness may become more noticeable in later stages of Parkinson's.

Infections: A variety of infections are associated with dizziness. Examples include:

COVID-19: You may feel dizziness and vertigo while you have or recover from COVID-19. The dizziness and vertigo may be associated with headaches and a loss of balance.

Other viral infections: Other viral infections, such as the flu or a cold, may also cause you to feel dizzy or lightheaded. These infections may be associated with dehydration as well.

Ear infection: An ear infection may lead to inflammation in your inner ear, causing dizziness and balance troubles. Ear infections are associated with both bacterial and viral causes.

Labyrinthitis and vestibular neuritis: Labyrinthitis and vestibular neuritis occur when specific nerves in your inner ear become inflamed. Triggers often include viral infections, but they can vary. Bacterial infections are more common in people with labyrinthitis than in people with vestibular neuritis.

In rare cases, a stroke, a malignant tumor, or another brain disorder can cause dizziness.

*Symptoms related to dizziness*

People who are dizzy may experience various sensations, including:

lightheadedness or faintness

a false sense of spinning

unsteadiness

a loss of balance

a feeling of floating

Sometimes, dizziness is accompanied by nausea, vomiting, or fainting. Seek emergency medical help if you have these symptoms for extended periods.

*When to call a doctor about dizziness*

It's important to call a doctor if you have repeated bouts of dizziness. Also, notify a doctor immediately if you experience sudden dizziness along with:

a head injury

a headache

neck stiffness

a high fever

ongoing vomiting

blurred vision

hearing loss

tinnitus

difficulty speaking

numbness or tingling

droopiness of the eye or mouth

loss of consciousness

chest pain

heart palpitations or a low heart rate

These symptoms could indicate a serious health problem, so it's important to seek medical attention as soon as possible. According to a 2021 Swedish study, 5% of people who used emergency services for dizziness had a time-critical medical issue.

Treatment for dizziness focuses on the underlying cause. In most cases, home remedies and medical treatments can help you manage the underlying cause. The following are potential treatments for the causes of dizziness:

Vertigo and benign positional vertigo (BPV): BPV, a common cause of vertigo, can often be resolved with the Epley maneuver. This exercise involves turning your head in specific ways to help alleviate symptoms. Surgery is typically not needed, but it's an option for people who can't manage their BPV otherwise.

Meniere's disease: This condition has no cure, but it may improve with medications, a healthful low-salt diet, antibiotic or corticosteroid injections, or ear surgery.

Acoustic neuroma: If the tumor grows, you may need radiation or surgery.

Dehydration: To help treat dehydration, drink plenty of fluids.

Migraine: Treatment for migraine attacks includes medications and lifestyle changes, such as learning to identify and avoid migraine triggers.

Alcohol: Drinking less alcohol may help you avoid dizziness from overconsumption.

Inner ear issues: You may be able to manage inner ear issues with medications or at-home exercises that help you maintain your balance.

Medications: If medications seem to be causing your dizziness, speak with a doctor about changing your medication or dose.

Sudden drop in blood pressure: Treatment for sudden low blood pressure depends on the cause or underlying condition, but it may involve adjusting your medications, exercising, or changing positions slowly when standing up.

Cardiomyopathy: This condition may be improved with medications or lifestyle changes such as quitting smoking and eating a heart-healthy diet.

Heart attack: A heart attack requires emergency treatment, which may include medications, oxygen therapy, or surgery.

Arrhythmia: Arrhythmia doesn't always require treatment. Healthy lifestyle choices, such as exercising and eating a balanced diet, can help you manage your symptoms. Heart medications are also available. Surgery is reserved for more serious cases.

Circulation problems: Circulation problems may improve with regular exercise, a heart-healthy diet, medications, or surgery.

Excessive exercise or heat exhaustion: Drinking plenty of fluids can help when dizziness is caused by excessive exercise or heat exhaustion.

Decrease in blood volume: Treatment for low blood volume focuses on restoring fluids through an intravenous (IV) line and treating underlying causes such as bleeding.

Anxiety disorders: Medications and anxiety-reducing techniques, such as therapy, can help with anxiety disorders.

Anemia: Iron supplements, medications, and eating a balanced diet can help treat anemia.

Hypoglycemia: If you have symptoms of hypoglycemia, try drinking fruit juice or soda or taking glucose tablets. For severely low blood glucose levels, you may need an injection of the hormone glucagon. Discover other emergency treatments for hypoglycemia.

Carbon monoxide poisoning: This condition requires immediate medical care. It may be treated with oxygen, a ventilator, and IV fluids.

Motion sickness: You can try ginger candy, aromatherapy, and over-the-counter (OTC) medications such as diphenhydramine (Benadryl) for motion sickness. Learn more about remedies for motion sickness.

Multiple sclerosis (MS): This condition currently has no cure, but physical therapy and medications may help with symptoms.

Parkinson's disease: Medications, surgery, and exercises may improve Parkinson's disease symptoms, though there is no cure at the moment.

Infections: Treatment will depend on the cause of the infection but will likely include hydration and rest.

COVID-19: Staying hydrated, resting, and doing balance exercises may help with dizziness that persists after a COVID-19 infection. If your symptoms get worse, it's important to have a doctor check for other underlying conditions.

Other viral infections: Hydration and rest are key to recovery. Antiviral medications are also available to help you manage conditions such as the flu. OTC medications such as decongestants and pain relievers can help treat a cold.

Ear infection: An ear infection may get better with rest and drinking fluids, or it may be treated with antibiotics.

Labyrinthitis and vestibular neuritis: Treatment often includes medications such as antidizziness medications, antihistamines, and antibiotics.

Stroke: You need emergency medical care for a stroke, which may include medications as well as surgery to repair and prevent internal bleeding.

Malignant tumor: Treatment may include surgery, radiation therapy, chemotherapy, or other medications.

Brain disorders: Treatments will vary depending on the disorder. Possible treatments include pain relievers, physical therapy, speech therapy, and surgery.

*Diagnosing the causes of dizziness*
A doctor can narrow down the cause of your dizziness by performing a physical examination. They'll ask you questions about your dizziness, including:

when it occurs

the situations where it occurs

how severe your symptoms are

which other symptoms occur with the dizziness

A doctor may also:

check your eyes and ears

perform a neurological exam

observe your posture

If the doctor suspects certain causes, including carbon monoxide poisoning, heart conditions, or a stroke, they may recommend a CT scan, an MRI, or another imaging test. You may also need additional tests. In some cases, a doctor can't determine the cause of dizziness.

Balance tests

A doctor or specialist may perform tests to check your balance. These tests look for problems with your inner ear that may affect your balance or cause dizziness. They include:

computerized dynamic posturography (CDP) test, where you try to maintain your balance while standing on a moving platform

Romberg test, which measures how well you keep your balance when standing with your eyes closed for 1 minute

electronystagmography (ENG) test, which involves a doctor placing sensors around your eyes and measuring your eye movements videonystagmography (VNG) test, in which you'll wear goggles and view light patterns so a doctor can measure your eye movements

rotary test, where goggles record your eye movements while you sit in a rotating, motorized chair


*Tests for vertigo*
If you have vertigo, the doctor may perform the following tests:

Dix-Hallpike maneuver, which involves turning your head and then switching quickly between lying down and sitting up so a doctor can check if you experience vertigo

vestibular evoked myogenic potentials (VEMP) test, in which a doctor looks for problems in your inner ear by playing sounds into earphones while you move your head and eyes

video head impulse test, which records your eye movements as you try to keep your eyes on a target while moving your head

Hearing tests

Hearing tests may also be performed for dizziness and balance issues. These tests may include:

otoacoustic emissions test, in which a small earphone plays sounds in your ear and a doctor measures the echoes that come back from your inner ear

tympanometry, in which a doctor blows air into your ear to evaluate the movement of your eardrum

electrocochleography, which tests the electrical activity of the cochlea (a hollow bone in the inner ear) using an electrode placed in the ear

Electrocochleography can help diagnose Meniere's disease.


Cardiac tests

Tests that can help a doctor diagnose cardiac causes of dizziness include the:

electrocardiogram (EKG), which they use to measure your heart's electrical activity echocardiogram, which is a type of ultrasound that reveals how well your heart works

stress test, where a doctor monitors your heart as you use a treadmill or perform another type of exercise

*Tips for managing dizziness*
Follow these tips if you have recurrent bouts of dizziness:

Sit or lie down immediately when you feel dizzy and rest until the dizziness goes away. This can prevent you from possibly losing your balance, which may lead to falling and serious injury.

Use a cane or walker for stability, if necessary.

Always use handrails when walking up or down stairs.

Try activities that can help improve your balance, such as yoga and tai chi.

Avoid moving or switching positions suddenly.

Avoid driving a car or operating heavy machinery if you frequently experience dizziness without warning.

Avoid caffeine, alcohol, and tobacco. Using these substances may trigger dizziness or make it worse.

Drink plenty of water and get sufficient sleep. Avoiding stressful situations may also be helpful.

If you suspect a medication is causing your dizziness, talk with your doctor about lowering the dose or switching to another medication.

Take an OTC medication such as meclizine (Antivert, Bonine) if you experience nausea along with dizziness. These medications may cause drowsiness, so do not use them when you need to be active or productive.

Rest in a cool place and drink water if your dizziness is caused by overheating or dehydration.

Always speak with a doctor if you're concerned about the frequency or severity of your dizziness. Most cases of dizziness clear up on their own once you treat the underlying cause. In rare cases, dizziness can be a symptom of a more serious health problem. Dizziness may result in complications related to fainting or a loss of balance. This can be especially dangerous when you're driving, operating heavy machinery, or climbing a ladder. Use caution if you feel an episode of dizziness coming on. If you become dizzy, stop driving immediately or find a safe place to steady yourself until the feeling passes.

## Complex Partial Seizures

A complex partial seizure is also known as a focal impaired awareness seizure or a focal onset impaired awareness seizure. This type of seizure starts in a single area of the brain. This area is usually, but not always, the temporal lobe of the brain. While it's most common in people with epilepsy, this type of seizure has been known to occur in people with cerebral palsy. It includes uncontrolled movement of limbs or other body parts. These seizures are usually very short, and the person having the seizure will be unaware of their surroundings. They may also become unconscious for a brief period of time.

Complex partial seizures and epilepsy

For those with epilepsy, this is the most common type of seizure. But while complex partial seizures are often related to epilepsy, this is not the only reason for someone to have seizures.

Symptoms of complex partial seizures

A complex partial seizure can have multiple possible symptoms. However, these symptoms may occur during one seizure and not another. Complex partial seizures normally only last a few minutes. Seizures beginning in the frontal lobe area of the brain are usually shorter than those that start in the temporal lobe area. Symptoms will often start abruptly, and the person experiencing the seizure may not know they have had one. The person may:

stare blankly or look like they're daydreaming

be unable to respond

wake from sleep suddenly

swallow, smack their lips, or otherwise move their mouth repetitively

pick at things like the air, clothing, or furniture

say words repetitively

scream, laugh, or cry

perform actions that can cause potential danger to themselves, like walking in front of moving cars or removing all or portions of their clothing

perform movements like they are riding a bicycle

be unaware, either partially or totally, of their surroundings

hallucinate

try to hurt themselves

experience confusion when the seizure ends

be unable to remember the seizure when it's over

Causes of complex partial seizures

While epilepsy is one of the most common causes, there are other conditions that can cause a complex partial seizure. Some of these conditions are:

psychological distress or trauma

neurologic conditions

extreme stress

anxiety and depression

autism

other medical conditions related to the brain

damage caused prior to birth

neurofibromatosis

Common triggers

A complex partial seizure can happen anytime and usually without much warning. They can even occur when the person is in the middle of an activity. Sometimes the person will have an aura right before having a complex partial seizure. An aura is also called a simple partial seizure. It can act as a warning signal that a bigger seizure is coming. There are some additional factors that can trigger a seizure, including:

flashing lights

low blood sugar

high fever

reactions to some medications

Diagnosing a complex partial seizure

Before deciding on treatment, a doctor will need to confirm that a person is having complex partial seizures. The doctor will need as many details as possible from the person having the seizures as well as from someone who has seen these episodes on a number of occasions. The doctor will need to know what happens before, during, and after each episode.

If a doctor suspects a complex partial seizure, they will usually order a diagnostic test to confirm. An electroencephalogram (EEG) may be done initially. However, the EEG will usually need to record a seizure to be accurate. Other tests that may be given to look for any potential cause of the seizures are a CT scan and an MRI. A blood test and neurological exam may be done as well. These may help the doctor find a cause (if there is a recognizable cause) without seeing an actual seizure while testing.

How are they treated and managed?

There are various types of treatment for complex partial seizures once the condition has been diagnosed. The following are some of the possible treatment options:

antiepileptic drugs (AEDs)

tiagabine hydrochloride (Gabitril), a new AED that shows promise in clinical trialsTrusted Source

stimulation of the vagus nerve

responsive neurostimulation

surgery

dietary changes

The type of treatment used is determined by the cause of the seizures, other medical conditions, and other factors.


Associated health conditions

A complex partial seizure can happen to anyone. However, there are some medical conditions that are more prone to these types of seizures. These medical conditions include:

epilepsy (most common)

cerebral palsy

infection in the brain

brain injury

tumor in the brain

stroke

some heart conditions

Sometimes a complex partial seizure will happen to someone without any known medical conditions. There is not always a cause that can be determined in some cases of complex partial seizures. Once diagnosed, seizures — including complex partial seizures — can be managed through a variety of treatment options. In some cases, children will outgrow the seizures. If you think that you or someone you know is having seizures, it's important to talk to a doctor for proper diagnosis and treatment. You should contact a medical professional immediately if someone you know is having a seizure and any of the following is true:

this is the person's first seizure

the seizure lasts more than five minutes

the person has a high fever

the person does not become conscious after the seizure is over

the person has diabetes

the person is or might be pregnant


## Are There Different Types of Epilepsy?

Your brain contains billions of nerve cells, also known as neurons. These neurons use electrical activity to communicate and send signals. If there's an abnormal change in this electrical activity, it can produce a seizure. Epilepsy is a condition in which seizures repeatedly occur.

Traditionally, epilepsy was defined as a type of disorder. It was sometimes referred to as an "epilepsy disorder." However, epilepsy is now officially known as a disease rather than a disorder. The classification of epilepsy types has also changed. This was done to help people better understand epilepsy and improve diagnosis.

New terminology for epilepsy and seizures

The International League Against Epilepsy (ILAE) is an organization that studies epilepsy. They publish reports that provide updated classifications of epilepsies and seizures that are agreed upon by the leading organizations. In 2005, epilepsy was defined as a brain disorder characterized by seizures. However, in 2014, the ILAE released an official reportTrusted Source changing the definition to "disease." According to the report, the term "disorder" suggests a disruption that isn't necessarily long-term. The word "disorder" could also diminish the seriousness of epilepsy and is often misunderstood. The ILAE stated that "disease" is a more accurate term to describe epilepsy. "Disease" generally implies more long-term disruptions.In 2017, the

ILAE published another report announcing new classifications of epilepsies and seizures. These guidelines introduced new terms and removed some older ones.

The new classification system categorized epilepsy according to its type of seizure. The goals of this new system include:

easier classification

easier, more accurate diagnosis

better guidance for medical and surgical treatments

These changes make it easier to understand and classify different epilepsies, as well as the seizures involved in each one.

## Types of epilepsy and symptoms

There are four types of epilepsies. Each type includes different types of seizures, which cause different symptoms and have different onset (begin in different parts of the brain). Identifying the type of seizure and where it begins in the brain guides treatment because medications used for one type can sometimes worsen another type. Epilepsy types include:

Focal epilepsy

Focal onset epilepsy involves focal seizures, or seizures that begin on one side of the brain. Focal epilepsies are common. About 60 percentTrusted Source of all types of epilepsy are focal. Seizures in this category include:

Simple focal seizures

A simple focal seizure can be similar to a seizure aura and it is sometimes called a seizure aura. You stay conscious and aware of your surroundings but sometimes unable to fully respond during the seizure. It might also cause:

muscle jerking

feeling of déjà vu

strange sensations, like odd smells

anxiety

hallucinations

Complex focal seizures

A complex focal seizure causes altered consciousness, but not necessarily complete loss of consciousness. Other symptoms include:

confusion

blank staring

repetitive movements, like blinking or gulping

A simple focal seizure can progress to a complex focal seizure. A simple or complex focal seizure that progresses to a generalized seizure is called a secondarily generalized seizure.

*Generalized epilepsy*
Generalized epilepsy involves generalized onset seizures. These seizures begin on both sides of the brain and cause impaired consciousness or loss of consciousness. Approximately 23 to 35 percent of epilepsies are generalized. It includes the following seizures:

Absence seizures

An absence seizure, formerly called a petit mal seizure, lasts for about 15 seconds and affects the whole brain. Symptoms include:

lack of awareness and lack of responsiveness while appearing conscious

suddenly stopping movement

appearance of daydreaming

confusion

slight muscle twitching

usually not remembering what happened during the seizure

Myoclonic seizures

Myoclonic seizures are brief, lasting a few seconds or less. You might have multiple myoclonic seizures within a short time. Other symptoms include:

staying fully or partially conscious

increase in muscle tone of some muscles

possible altered sensations, such as a sensation of an electric shock

Tonic-clonic seizures

Generalized tonic-clonic (GTC) seizures were previously called grand mal seizures. Symptoms include:

loss of consciousness

falls

muscle stiffening (tonic phase) and jerking (clonic phase)

crying out

Tonic seizures

A tonic seizure causes muscle stiffening, but it doesn't have a clonic phase. You might stay conscious or experience a brief change in awareness.

Clonic seizures

A clonic seizure causes muscle spasms and jerking for several minutes. You may lose awareness.

Atonic seizures

Also called drop attacks, atonic seizures cause a sudden loss of muscle tone. This might cause:

staying aware or briefly losing consciousness

head dropping

slumping

falls

injury due to fall

Combined generalized and focal epilepsy

If both generalized onset and focal onset seizures occur, it's called combined generalized and focal epilepsy. This type of epilepsy causes a combination of various seizures, including one or more of:

generalized tonic-clonic seizures

myoclonic seizures

absence seizures

tonic seizures

atonic seizures

The seizures can occur together or separately. One type of seizure can occur more frequently than others. The exact symptoms depend on the seizures involved.

Unknown if generalized or focal epilepsy

Sometimes, it's not possible to determine the type of seizures. This might happen if there isn't enough medical information to classify the seizure onset. One example is an electroencephalogram (EEG) with normal results. In this case, the epilepsy is categorized as "unknown" until there is more information.

What are epilepsy syndromes?

An epilepsy syndrome refers to a set of medical features that usually appear together. This includes seizure types, along with:

age when seizures typically start

EEG results

common triggers

genetic factors

outlook

response to antiepileptic drugs

other symptoms, such as physical or cognitive problems

This is different from an epilepsy type. An epilepsy type only indicates the types of seizures. An epilepsy syndrome describes the types of seizures (and therefore, epilepsy type), plusother characteristics. To date, there are more than 30 known epilepsy syndromes. Examples include:

Dravet syndrome

childhood absence epilepsy

gelastic epilepsy

Laundau Kleffner syndrome

Lennox-Gastaut syndrome

Doose syndrome (myoclonic astatic epilepsy)

West syndrome (infantile spasms)

What types of epilepsy syndromes are most common in children

Epilepsy syndromes often appear in childhood. The most common childhood syndromes include:

benign rolandic epilepsy

childhood idiopathic occipital epilepsy

childhood absence epilepsy

juvenile myoclonic epilepsy

How types of epilepsy are diagnosed

A doctor will use several tests to determine what type of epilepsy you might have. These include:

Physical exam. A doctor will check if you have physical problems in addition to your seizures. They'll also test your motor skills.

Medical history. Since epilepsy is often inherited, a doctor will want to learn more about your family's history.

Blood tests. Your doctor will test markers that might be related to seizures. Examples include low blood sugar or inflammatory markers.

Neuropsychological exam. A specialist will test your cognition, speech, and memory. This helps them determine where the seizures are happening in your brain and if there are other associated problems.

Electroencephalogram. An electroencephalogram (EEG) measures your brain's electrical activity and it can help identify where the seizure is starting, and whether it is focal onset or generalized onset.

Imaging tests. An imaging tests lets your doctor check for lesions or structural abnormalities that may be causing seizures. Examples include a computerized tomography (CT) scan or magnetic resonance imaging (MRI).

*How are different types of epilepsy and epilepsy syndromes treated?*

An epilepsy syndrome is treated based on its clinical features. This includes the type of epilepsy and seizures involved. Treatment may include:

Antiepileptic drugs. Antiepileptic drugs (AEDs) reduce the frequency or severity of seizures. The type of seizure will determine the most effective option.

Surgery. Surgery for epilepsy involves cutting or removing part of the brain where seizures are happening and it can control some types of epilepsy.

High-fat diet. If AEDs don't work or you can't get surgery, your doctor might suggest a high-fat, low-carb diet for certain types of epilepsy. This might include a ketogenic diet or modified Atkins diet.

Vagus nerve stimulation. A small electrical device is implanted under the skin to stimulate the vagus nerve, which controls some of your brain activity. The device helps control certain seizures by stimulating the nerve.

Types of epilepsy are classified by the types of seizures involved. The main epilepsy types include focal onset epilepsy, generalized onset epilepsy, combined generalized and focal epilepsy, and unknown onset. A doctor can use various tests to determine what type of epilepsy you might have. This may include a physical exam, blood tests, imaging scans, and an EEG. Depending on the type, epilepsy might be treated with drugs, surgery, vagus nerve stimulation, and/or a high-fat diet.

# CONCLUSION

Generalized seizures affect your whole brain. Focal, or partial seizures, affect only one part of your brain. A mild seizure may be difficult to recognize. It may only last a few seconds, and you may remain awake while it happens. Stronger seizures can cause spasms and uncontrollable muscle twitches. They can last from a few seconds to several minutes and may cause confusion or loss of consciousness. Afterward, you may have no memory of a seizure happening.There's currently no cure for epilepsy, but it can be managed with medications and other strategies.